Cognitive Stimulation Therapy

and

Therapeutic Exercise

- A Primer

Olaide Oluwole-Sangoseni, PhD, DPT, MSc

AOS PROVIDENT WELLNESS OUTREACH

PREFACE

To God be the glory!

This manual introduces students to the concept of multicomponent therapeutic intervention using cognitive stimulation therapy and therapeutic exercise in physical therapy.

First Edition, 2020

ACKNOWLEDGMENTS

Many thanks to Jill Heitzman, PT, DPT, PhD, for her helpful suggestions for the first manuscript.

My gratitude to my dedicated editor, Opeoluwa Sangoseni, Cert. CST, for her helpful review of content and tireless edits of the many iterations of this manuscript.

TABLE OF CONTENTS

Introduction

Therapeutic exercise or exercise therapy is a specific, intensive regimen of structured physical activities designed and prescribed to restore or maintain normal musculoskeletal functioning, facilitate recovery, or reduce pain.[1,2]

Is exercise the same as physical activity?

- Physical activity is defined as any bodily movement involving the skeletal muscles. It requires significant energy expenditure above the baseline utility and is measured in metabolic energy equivalent or MET. 1MET is 3.5ml/kg/min of O_2.
- Exercise is a planned, structured, purposeful, and repetitive movement aimed at improving or maintaining physical fitness. Exercise is a subcategory of physical activity.
- Physical fitness is the ability to perform activities of daily living with alertness and agility, enjoy daily leisure tasks, or handle day-to-day stressors appropriately and reflexively. Measurable physical fitness components include aerobics, balance, coordination, flexibility, strength, and power.

Benefits of Exercise

Regardless of age, physical activity improves the function, response, and performance (fitness) of the cardiovascular, pulmonary, neurological, and musculoskeletal systems.[1-4] Therapeutic exercise significantly enhances muscular strength, endurance, and flexibility. It produces beneficial physiological changes in the skeletal joints and body composition. There is much empirical evidence of the positive impact of exercise on cardiopulmonary endurance on a short and long term basis.

Research suggests that exercise compares favorably to antidepressant medications as a first-line treatment for mild to moderate depression and has also been shown to improve depressive symptoms when used as an adjunct to medications.[2] Exercise enables physiological changes that lead to improved sleep

1

and metabolism and the release of central nervous system neurotransmitters, serotonin, and endogenous opioid neuropeptides hormones, endorphins. Other associated physical changes to the brain include increased volume, blood flow, and an overall boost in neural functioning.[1,5]

According to the World Health Organization (WHO), physical inactivity is the fourth leading cause of death globally.[6] Further, physical inactivity of a level below recommendation for optimal health promotion, disease prevention, and wellness lead to premature death. Physical inactivity is a significant predisposing factor for many non-communicable chronic disease conditions that impact older adults' functional mobility and well-being.

Therapeutic exercise is a critical interventional approach used by physical therapists regardless of practice setting. According to the American Physical Therapy Association, physical therapists (PTs) are movement experts who improve quality of life through prescribed exercise, hands-on care, and patient education.[3] PTs holistically care for people of all ages who want to become healthier and prevent future problems. PTs accomplish this through examination, and subsequent development of a specialized treatment plan intends to improve the patient's ability to move optimally, reduce or manage pain, restore function, and prevent disability. PTs practice in a wide range of settings, including hospitals, outpatient clinics, people's homes, schools, sports and fitness facilities, workplaces, and nursing homes.[4] PTs are movement/exercise experts across the lifespan. PTs and physical therapist assistants promote physical activity/exercise. They are clinical/health educators, health and wellness advocates, and patient partners in healthful living.

Cognitive Stimulation Therapy

In the United Kingdom, the National Institute of Health and Care Excellence (NICE-SCIE Guidance, 2006) recommended that individuals diagnosed with mild or moderate dementia should participate in a structured group cognitive stimulation program conducted by skilled personnel regardless of whether or not they were placed on an anti-dementia medication regimen.[7,8] Similar recommendations have been made both here in the United States and in other countries.

What is Cognitive Stimulation Therapy - CST?

Cognitive stimulation therapy (CST) is a nonpharmacological structured group treatment first developed in the United Kingdom for people with mild to moderate dementia.[9] This internationally recognized therapy approach is an adaptation of Reality Orientation. The treatment consists of 14 sessions with an array of activities, tasks, and discussions focused on augmentation of cognitive and social functioning. The sessions focus on actively engaging people with dementia in an optimal sociocultural learning environment that provides the psychosocial benefits of being part of a group.[10]

Key Principles of CST

- Orientating people sensitively / when appropriate
- Information processing and opinion rather than factual knowledge, known as implicit learning
- Multi-sensory stimulation
- Flexible activities to cater to the group's needs and abilities
- Using reminiscence (as an aid to here-and-now)
- Building/strengthening relationships

Components of CST

1.	Physical games	8.	Being creative
2.	Sound	9.	Categorizing objects
3.	Childhood	10.	Orientation
4.	Food	11.	Using money
5.	Current affairs	12.	Number games
6.	Faces/scenes	13.	Word games
7.	Word association	14.	Team quiz

Benefits of CST

According to the developers of the program and empirical research from others' review of the program, the CST program maximizes an individual's potential by:

- facilitating engagement through active learning,
- stimulating development of new ideas, thoughts, and associations,
- increasing orientation by the focus on cognitive strength,
- utilizing reminiscence sensitivity,
- utilizing triggers to improve concentration and recall,
- promoting consistency and continuity session to session using repetition
- stimulating language and executive function skills
- promoting person-centered environment with respect and involvement
- promoting choice-making, relationship-building, and fun

Comparing CST and Exercise Therapy

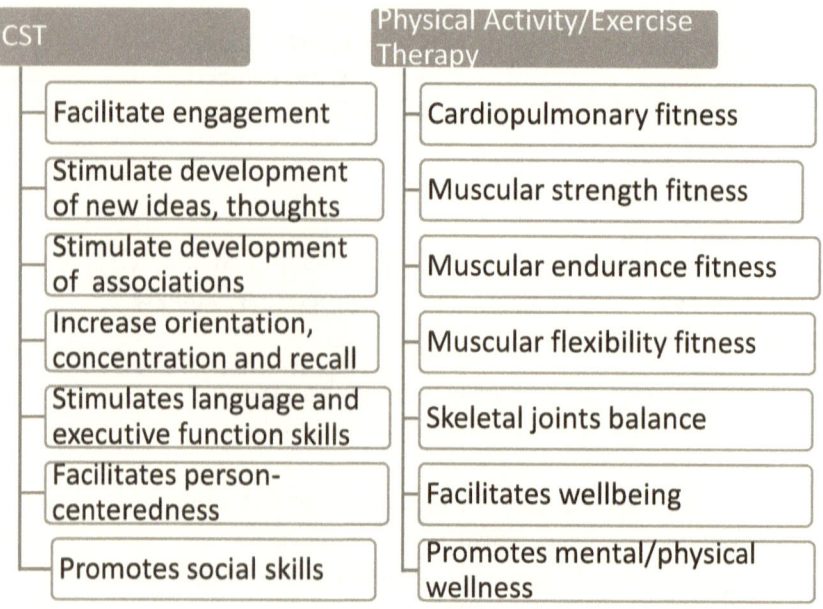

CST program consists of:

- 14 sessions, each of 45 minutes (twice weekly for seven weeks)
- Participants asked to give a group name
- Reality Orientation board
- Two facilitators
- Sessions begin with a warm-up exercise
- Bridging between sessions, consistency in time, place, participants and facilitators
- Presenting sessions in a fun and stimulating way

Need for Integrating Cognitive Stimulation Therapy and Therapeutic Exercise

The APTA Choose Wisely Campaign states, "Don't prescribe under-dosed strength training programs for older adults. Instead, match the frequency, intensity, and duration of exercise to the individual's abilities and goals."[11]

However, despite the agreed benefits of exercise therapy, adherence remains a challenge among people of all ages, especially among older adults.[12-16] Experts have suggested that exercise therapy program must be prescribed with adherence factors to ensure participation that leads to expected benefits. Recommendations for facilitating adherence include:

- Using motivational health interview to understand and identify needs to create a patient-partner

- Shared decision-making on person-centered wellness goals

- Ensuring ownership by fostering autonomy and respect as defined in cultural context

- Positively reinforcing and incentivizing tangible and intangible efforts

- Utilizing the power of peer-to-peer motivation

Who is an Older Adult?

Old age is an increase in chronological age whereby the cut-off is defined in the environment's context. For example, The World Health Organization classifies older adults as individuals age 50 years and above. Whereas, in the United States, for socioeconomic and health policy reasons, older adults are individuals 65 years and older in many circumstances. The AARP – a United States-based nonprofit advocacy organization for older Americans establishes older adults 50 years and above. At the state level, old age definition varies. For example, in the state of Missouri, old age is 60 years and above.

A note about Cognition and Physical Aging

Even though there are normal physiological changes that occur with increasing age, most exercise recommendations apply to individuals of all ages. The fundamental principles of exercise therapy – the principle of overload, reversibility, and specificity - apply to all individuals, especially older adults.

Exercise Dose-Response for Normal Aging in older adults

Thus to obtain gains in flexibility, balance, proprioception, or strength, exercise therapy must follow the following recommendation at the minimum: frequency of 2 - 3 days per week at moderate intensity (MET) defined 60-70% 1 RM for 30-60minutes per day or light intensity at 40-50% of 1RM for 20-30minutes each day. The rate of perceived exertion (RPE) of 14 – 16/20; 4-6/10

Multicomponent exercise therapy is best suited for older adults with mild to moderate cognitive impairment.[13,18] Dual-tasking that incorporates cognitive training and motor skill training has been shown in many research to be more effective in improving motor performance than single task repetitive training. Cognitive-Dual-Task Training has been shown to increase neuropriming for enhanced benefits of therapeutic exercise.[18-22] Although more research is needed in this area, multimodal exercise has been shown to improve attention, executive function, processing speed for transfer and retrieval of contextual information, mainly from short term into long term memory.

CST Structure with Physical Therapy

Activity Promotes Mobility

CST-Exercise Therapy is what I called an "activity that facilitates mobility" session. It begins with a holistic physical therapy screening, which establishes a baseline for exercise capability and uses vital signs[17] as exercise readiness and response measures.

Baseline Screen before CST- Exercise Therapy Session

- Screen with the Rapid Geriatric Assessment (RGA)
- Blood pressure (BP): 90/60 mmHg - 120/80 mmHg
- Breathing (RR): 12 - 18 breaths per minute
- Pulse (HR): 60 - 100 beats per minute
- Temperature: 97.8°F - 99.1°F (36.5°C - 37.3°C); average 98.6°F (37°C)
- Oxygen Saturation (SpO_2): 96 – 98% (careful to factor machine or instrument error in persons with darker skin or with nail polish)
- Assess handgrip strength
- Timed-Up and Go (TUG): <13.2 secs

Sample CST Structure with Physical Therapy

- Welcome

- Take Vital signs – BP, HR, RR, SpO_2

- Theme song – related to one of the 14 components

  - Exercise/Movement Therapy – Warm-up

- Orientation discussion

  - Exercise/Movement Therapy

- Current Affairs

  - Exercise/Movement Therapy

- Theme song

  - Exercise/Movement Therapy – Cooldown

- Reminders for next sessions

- Farewell

Sample Standard CST Program Components – Weeks 1 – 7

1. Physical Games – softball, bowling

2. Sound – sing-along; play music from their time – name the instruments, artists, dress code, etc.

3. Childhood – where did you go on vacation when you were a child? Were you named after someone? – a saint, a relative, a family friend

4. Current Affairs – what do you think of reality shows? Or social media? Or cell phone? What do you think of politicians? Discuss recent news headlines.

5. Faces/Scenes - what do these people have in common? How are they different? Who would you rather be? Teacher, PT, RN, firefighter, etc.

6. Food – what is your favorite food? Fruits, veggies, drinks, etc.

7. Word Association – apple ---; fruit ----

Sample Standard CST Program Components – Weeks 8 – 14

8. Being Creative – what is your hobby?

9. Categorizing objects – 3 things found in a grocery store; or in a kitchen; or musical instrument, clothing; colors, animals, etc.

10. Orientation – Is anyone's birthday around now? Does it feel hotter or wetter? Do you think this weather is typical for spring or summer or winter?

11. Using money – what can you buy today for $1 or $5?

12. Number games – Count by 2s, 3s, 4s

13. Word games – e.g. Hangman

14. Team quiz – what was your occupation?

How Does It Look? CST and Exercise Therapy

CST/PT: Week 1 – Hobbies/Dual-task training

- Welcome – Take Vital signs BP, HR, RR, SpO$_2$

- Theme song – related to one of the 14 components

    - Exercise/Movement Therapy – Warm-up
      (Marching in place to the beat of "Cheers" ~3 min)

- Orientation discussion – discuss different hobbies

    - Exercise/Movement Therapy

    - Room search activity requiring squatting (legs)
      and reaching (arms)

- Theme song – "Cheers."

    - Exercise/Movement Therapy – Cool Down

        - Full Body Relaxation Technique (feeling
          your neck, arms, hands, back, legs, feet)

        - Deep Breathing Exercises to slow heart
          rate

- Reminders for next sessions

- Farewell

Cognitive Stimulation Therapy and Exercise Therapy- A Primer

CST/PT: Week 1 – Hobbies (Alternative) /Dual-task training

- Welcome – Take Vital signs BP, HR, RR, SpO_2
- Theme song – related to hobbies
- Exercise/Movement Therapy – Warm-up (Marching in place to the beat of "Cheers" ~3 min)
- Orientation discussion – discuss different hobbies
    - Exercise/Movement Therapy: Duck Chair Goose
- Theme song – "Cheers"
    - Exercise/Movement Therapy – Cool Down
        - Full Body Relaxation Technique (feeling your neck, arms, hands, back, legs, feet)
        - Deep Breathing Exercises to slow heart rate
- Reminders for next sessions
- Farewell

CST/PT: Week 2 – Childhood/Dual-task training

- Welcome – Take Vital signs BP, HR, RR, SpO$_2$

- Theme song – related to one of the 14 components

    - Exercise/Movement Therapy – Warm-up
      (Marching in place to the beat of "Cheers" ~3 min)

- Orientation discussion- what is today's date? Who's the president? Where are you? What city do you live in? Why are you here? What is your name?

- Exercise/Movement Therapy

- Childhood- pick a "recess" type game, e.g., Red light/green light, musical chairs, TV tag, etc.

    - Ask questions about their childhood during the game (e.g., When they are "frozen" or on "red light," etc.)

    - Where were you born? When were you born? Where did you grow up?

- Exercise/Movement Therapy – Cool Down

    - Full Body Relaxation Technique (feeling your neck, arms, hands, back, legs, feet)

    - Deep Breathing Exercises to slow heart rate

- Reminders for next sessions

- Farewell

CST/PT: Week 3 or 4 – Current Affairs/Dual-task training

- Welcome – Take Vital signs BP, HR, RR, SpO$_2$

- Theme song – related to one of the 14 components

    - Exercise/Movement Therapy – Warm-up
      (Marching in place to the beat of "Cheers" ~3 min)

- Orientation discussion- what is today's date? Who's the president? Where are you? What city do you live in? Why are you here? What is your name?

- Exercise/Movement Therapy

- Current affairs- name that celebrity

- Cooldown- Review most recent news headlines

- Exercise/Movement Therapy – Cool Down

    - Full Body Relaxation Technique (feeling your neck, arms, hands, back, legs, feet)

    - Deep Breathing Exercises to slow heart rate

- Reminders for next sessions

- Farewell

CST/PT: Week 5 – Faces/Roles/Scenes/Dual-task training

- Welcome – Take Vital signs BP, HR, RR, SpO$_2$

- Theme song – related to one of the 14 components

- Exercise/Movement Therapy – Warm-up (Marching in place to the beat of "Macarena" ~3 min)

- Orientation discussion

    - What is today's date? Who's the president? Where are you? What city do you live in? Why are you here? What is your name?

- Exercise/Movement Therapy

    - Sit to stands –They say who the person is and place them in the correct category.

- Exercise/Movement Therapy – Cool Down

    - Full Body Relaxation Technique

    - Deep Breathing Exercises to slow heart rate

- Reminders for next sessions

- Farewell

!LIGHTBULB:

George Washington – presidents
Babe Ruth – sports
Cary Grant – actor/actress
Julie Andrews – actor/actress
Bill Clinton – presidents
Michael Jordan – sports
Wayne Gretzky – sports
Marilyn Monroe – actor/actress
Abraham Lincoln – presidents
Florence Henderson – actor/actress

CST/PT: Week 6 – Foods/Dual-task training

- Welcome – Take Vital signs BP, HR, RR, SpO$_2$

- Theme song – related to one of the 14 components

  - Exercise/Movement Therapy – Warm-up
    (Marching in place to "Macarena" song)

- Orientation discussion- Who's the president? What city do you live in?

- Group circle and toss a beach ball, then name something within the category before passing it along to the next person

- Food groups, Pizza toppings, Sodas, Desserts, Types of cuisines (culture-wise, Favorite food, Fruits, Veggies, etc

- Exercise/Movement Therapy – Cool Down

  - Full Body Relaxation Technique

- Reminders for next sessions

- Farewell

CST/PT: Week 6 – Foods/Dual-task training

- Name types of cheese while throwing or passing a ball

- Balance progression with ball toss while doing word association

- Standing - positions to progress through with each category:

    - Start with a normal stance

    - Feet together

    - Eyes closed with/without throwing a ball

!LIGHTBULB:

- Food categories:
    - Cheese
        - Gouda
        - Whiz
        - Cake
    - Nuts
        - Cashew
        - Almond
        - Pecan

CST/PT: Week 7 – Categorizing Things/Dual-task training

- Balance progression with ball toss while doing word association

- Dual-task training

- Positioning to progress through with each category:

    - Normal stance

    - Feet together

    - Tandem with R leg in front

    - Tandem with L leg in front

!LIGHTBULB

- Sports Balls/Objects
- Colors
- Musicians/Music Genres

Suggested Music Playlist

These dance songs are in no specific order of preference

1. I know who I am – Sinach
2. Diamonds on the Soles of Her Shoes – Paul Simon
3. Single Ladies – Beyonce
4. Wavin' Flag – K'naan
5. Uptown Funk – Bruno Mars
6. Every Praise (radio edit) – Hezekiah Walker
7. Man in the Mirror – Micahel Jackson
8. Macarena – Los del Rio
9. Forever and Ever, Amen – Randy Travis
10. Achy Breaky Heart – Billy Ray Cyrus
11. I Wanna Dance with Somebody (Who Loves Me) – Whitney Houston
12. Girls Just Want to Have Fun – Cyndi Lauper
13. 9 to 5 - Dolly Parton
14. Me Myself And I – De La Soul
15. Push It – Salt N Pepa
16. Happy – Pharell Williams
17. You Can Call Me Al – Paul Simon
18. The Happiness of Having You – Charley Pride
19. Ring of Fire – Johnny Cash
20. We Are Family – Sisters Sledge
21. Stayin Alive – Bee Gees
22. I Will Survive – Gloria Gaynor
23. Lean on Me – Bill Withers
24. That's The Way I Like It – KC & Sunshine
25. Twist and Shout – The Beatles
26. Run, Run, Rudolph – Chuck Berry
27. Uptown Funk – Bruno Mars
28. La Bamba – Los Lobos
29. Karma Chameleon – Boy Gorge
30. Break My Stride - Matthew Wilder

References

1. Barker K, Eickmeyer S. Therapeutic Exercise. Med Clin North Am. 2020 Mar;104(2):189-198. doi: 10.1016/j.mcna.2019.10.003. Epub 2019 Dec 16. PMID: 32035563.

2. Siciliano G, Schirinzi E, Simoncini C, Ricci G. Exercise therapy in muscle diseases: open issues and future perspectives. Acta Myol. 2019;38(4):233-238. Published 2019 Dec 1. Available at https://www.ncbi.nlm.nih.gov/pmc/articles/PMC6955631/

3. Carek PJ, Laibstain SE, Carek SM. Exercise for the treatment of depression and anxiety. Int J Psychiatry Med. 2011;41(1):15-28. doi: 10.2190/PM.41.1.c. PMID: 21495519.

4. American Physical Therapy Association. Becoming a PT. Available at https://www.apta.org/your-career/careers-in-physical-therapy/becoming-a-pt

5. Codella R, Terruzzi I, Luzi L. Sugars, exercise and health. J Affect Disord. 2017 Dec 15;224:76-86. doi: 10.1016/j.jad.2016.10.035. Epub 2016 Oct 27. PMID: 27817910.

6. Kohl HW 3rd, Craig CL, Lambert EV, Inoue S, Alkandari JR, Leetongin G, Kahlmeier S; Lancet Physical Activity Series Working Group. The pandemic of physical inactivity: global action for public health. Lancet. 2012 Jul 21;380(9838):294-305. doi: 10.1016/S0140-6736(12)60898-8. PMID: 22818941.

7. Spector A, Thorgrimsen L, Woods B, Royan L, Davies S, Butterworth M and Orrell M. Efficacy of an evidence-based cognitive stimulation therapy programme for people with dementia: Randomised Controlled Trial. British J Psychiatry 2003;183: 248-254.

8. National Institute for Health and Clinical Excellence. Dementia: supporting people with dementia and their carers in health and social care. 2006 NICE clinical guideline 42. www.nice.org.uk/guidance/cg42

9. Woods B, Aguirre E, Spector AE, Orrell M. Cognitive stimulation to improve cognitive functioning in people with dementia. Cochrane Database Syst Rev. 2012 Feb 15;(2):CD005562. doi: 10.1002/14651858.CD005562.pub2. PMID: 22336813.

10. Cheung, G. Peri Ki .Cognitive stimulation therapy: A New Zealand pilot. Auckland: Te Pou o Te Whakaaro Nui. 2014

11. American Physical Therapy Association. Choosing Wisely. ABIM Foundation. Available at https://www.choosingwisely.org/clinician-lists/american-physical-therapy-association-under-dosed-strength-training-for-older-adults/ December 28, 2020

12. Martínez-Velilla N, Casas-Herrero A, Zambom-Ferraresi F, et al. Effect of Exercise Intervention on Functional Decline in Very Elderly Patients During Acute Hospitalization: A Randomized Clinical Trial [published correction appears in JAMA Intern Med. 2019 Jan 1;179(1):127]. JAMA Intern Med. 2019;179(1):28-36. doi:10.1001/jamainternmed.2018.4869

13. Casas-Herrero A, Anton-Rodrigo I, Zambom-Ferraresi F, et al. Effect of a multicomponent exercise programme (VIVIFRAIL) on functional capacity in frail community elders with cognitive decline: study protocol for a randomized multicentre control trial. Trials. 2019;20(1):362. Published 2019 Jun 17. doi:10.1186/s13063-019-3426-0

14. Sáez de Asteasu ML, Martínez-Velilla N, Zambom-Ferraresi F, et al. Assessing the impact of physical

exercise on cognitive function in older medical patients during acute hospitalization: Secondary analysis of a randomized trial. PLoS Med. 2019;16(7):e1002852. Published 2019 Jul 5. doi:10.1371/journal.pmed.1002852

15. Taylor D. Physical activity is medicine for older adults. Postgrad Med J. 2014 Jan;90(1059):26-32. doi: 10.1136/postgradmedj-2012-131366. Epub 2013 Nov 19. PMID: 24255119; PMCID: PMC3888599.

16. Billot M, Calvani R, Urtamo A, Sánchez-Sánchez JL, Ciccolari-Micaldi C, Chang M, Roller-Wirnsberger R, Wirnsberger G, Sinclair A, Vaquero-Pinto N, Jyväkorpi S, Öhman H, Strandberg T, Schols JMGA, Schols AMWJ, Smeets N, Topinkova E, Michalkova H, Bonfigli AR, Lattanzio F, Rodríguez-Mañas L, Coelho-Júnior H, Broccatelli M, D'Elia ME, Biscotti D, Marzetti E, Freiberger E. Preserving Mobility in Older Adults with Physical Frailty and Sarcopenia: Opportunities, Challenges, and Recommendations for Physical Activity Interventions. Clin Interv Aging. 2020 Sep 16;15:1675-1690. doi: 10.2147/CIA.S253535. PMID: 32982201; PMCID: PMC7508031.

17. Ostchega Y, Porter KS, Hughes J, Dillon CF, Nwankwo T. Resting pulse rate reference data for children, adolescents, and adults: United States, 1999-2008. Natl Health Stat Report. 2011;(41):1-16.

18. Bonnechère B, Bier JC, Van Hove O, Sheldon S, Samadoulougou S, Kirakoya-Samadoulougou F, Klass M. Age-Associated Capacity to Progress When Playing Cognitive Mobile Games: Ecological Retrospective Observational Study. JMIR Serious Games. 2020 Jun 12;8(2):e17121. doi: 10.2196/17121. PMID: 32530432; PMCID: PMC7320308.

19. Bula C. Physical activity and cognitive function in older persons. Swiss Sport Exerc Med 2016; 64(2):14-18.

20. Morris JK, Vidoni ED, Johnson DK, Van Sciver A, Mahnken JD, Honea RA, Wilkins HM, Brooks WM, Billinger SA, Swerdlow RH, Burns JM.Aerobic exercise for Alzheimer's disease: A randomized controlled pilot trial. PLoS One. 2017;12(2):e0170547. Published 2017 Feb 10. doi:10.1371/journal.pone.0170547

21. Zhang W, Low LF, Gwynn JD, Clemson L. Interventions to Improve Gait in Older Adults with Cognitive Impairment: A Systematic Review. J Am Geriatr Soc. 2019;67(2):381-391. doi:10.1111/jgs.15660

22. Lam FM, Huang MZ, Liao LR, Chung RC, Kwok TC, Pang MY. Physical exercise improves strength, balance, mobility, and endurance in people with cognitive impairment and dementia: a systematic review. J Physiother. 2018;64(1):4-15. doi:10.1016/j.jphys.2017.12.001

Appendix A

Rapid Geriatric Assessment*

*There is no copyright on these screening tools and they may be incorporated into the Electronic Health Record without permission and at no cost.

The Simple "FRAIL" Questionnaire Screening Tool
(3 or greater = frailty; 1 or 2 = prefrail)

Fatigue: Are you fatigued?
Resistance: Cannot walk up one flight of stairs?
Aerobic: Cannot walk one block?
Illnesses: Do you have more than 5 illnesses?
Loss of weight: Have you lost more than 5% of your weight in the last 6 months?

From Morley JE, Vellas B, Abellan van Kan G, et al. J Am Med Dir Assoc 2013;14:392-397.

Table I: SARC-F Screen for Sarcopenia

Component	Question	Scoring
Strength	How much difficulty do you have in lifting and carrying 10 pounds?	None = 0 Some = 1 A lot or unable = 2
Assistance in walking	How much difficulty do you have walking across a room?	None = 0 Some = 1 A lot, use aids, or unable = 2
Rise from a chair	How much difficulty do you have transferring from a chair or bed?	None = 0 Some = 1 A lot or unable without help = 2
Climb stairs	How much difficulty do you have climbing a flight of ten stairs?	None = 0 Some = 1 A lot or unable = 2
Falls	How many times have you in the last year?	None = 0 fallen 1-3 falls = 1 4 or more falls = 2

From Malmstrom TK, Morley JE. J Frailty and Aging 2013;2:55-6.

SNAQ (Simplified Nutritional Assessment Questionnaire)

My appetite is
a. very poor
b. poor
c. average
d. good
e. very good

Food tastes
a. very bad
b. bad
c. average
d. good
e. very good

When I eat
a. I feel full after eating only a few mouthfuls
b. I feel full after eating about a third of a meal
c. I feel full after eating over half a meal
d. I feel full after eating most of the meal
e. I hardly ever feel full

Normally I eat
a. less than one meal a day
b. one meal a day
c. two meals a day
d. three meals a day
e. more than three meals a day

From Wilson et al. Am J Clin Nutr 2005;82:1074-81.

Miscellaneous
Are you constipated? Y/N
Do you have worrisome incontinence? Y/N
Do you have an advanced directive? Y/N

Rapid Cognitive Screen (RCS)

1. Please remember these five objects. I will ask you what they are later. [Read each object to patient using approx. 1 second intervals.]
   Apple   Pen   Tie   House   Car
2. [Give patient pencil and the blank sheet with clock face.] This is a clock face. Please put in the hour markers and the time at ten minutes to eleven o'clock. [2 pts/hr markers ok; 2 pts/time correct]
3. What were the five objects I asked you to remember? [1 pt/ea]
4. I'm going to tell you a story. Please listen carefully because afterwards, I'm going to ask you about it.

Jill was a very successful stockbroker. She made a lot of money on the stock market. She then met Jack, a devastatingly handsome man. She married him and had three children. They lived in Chicago. She then stopped work and stayed at home to bring up her children. When they were teenagers, she went back to work. She and Jack lived happily ever after.
What state did she live in? [1 pt]

From Malmstrom TK, Voss VB, Cruz-Oliver DM et al. J Nutr Health Aging 2015;19:741-744.

www.ingramcontent.com/pod-product-compliance
Lightning Source LLC
Chambersburg PA
CBHW030553220526
45463CB00007B/3072